Living with Osteoporosis

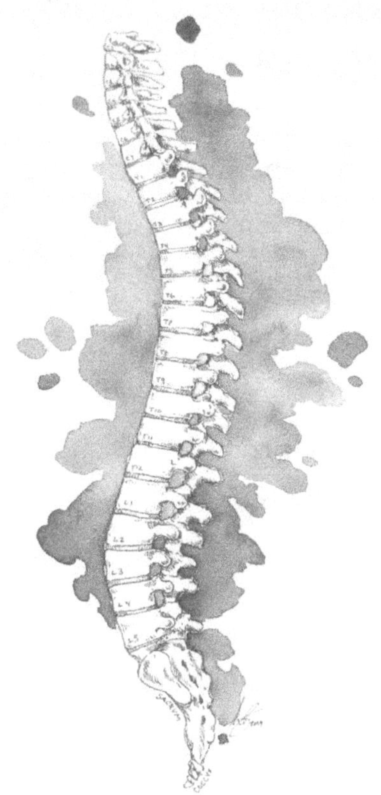

The Forgotten Disease and its Impact on Aging Populations

Anna Brown

TABLE OF CONTENTS

INTRODUCTION

Why Osteoporosis is a Concern for Aging Populations

Osteoporosis is a chronic disease that damages the bones and makes them fragile. When the body either loses too much bone tissue or does not produce enough new bone tissue, it results in this condition. Bones become brittle and prone to fractures as a result.

Any bone in the body can develop osteoporosis, but the hip, spine, and wrist are the most often affected. Because bone density gradually declines with age, leaving people more prone to fractures, osteoporosis is a serious problem for aging populations.

In addition, older persons frequently have additional health issues such as hormone imbalances, chronic inflammation, and dietary deficiencies that might raise the risk of osteoporosis. Additionally, bone loss may exacerbate in elderly persons because they may be less physically active.

Osteoporosis is a substantial problem for aging populations because of all of these reasons, making prevention and treatment crucial to preserving older persons' independence and health.

CHAPTER ONE: UNDERSTANDING OSTEOPOROSIS

What is Osteoporosis?

Minerals, mostly calcium salts, are what make up bone and are held together by strong collagen fibers. Known as cortical or compact bone, this thick, hard outer layer of our bones is seen on X-rays. Trabecular bone, a softer, spongier bone mesh with a honeycomb-like structure, is included inside this.

The bone is a dynamic, living tissue that is continually regenerating. Osteoclasts, which break down old bone tissue, are then replaced by osteoblasts, which create new bone tissue. At various times during our lifetimes, the ratio of bone production to bone resorption fluctuates.

Young children and adolescents experience a rapid bone-growth rate. Our bones can enlarge and become denser as a result. By our mid- to late-20s, bone density peaks. After then, the production of new bone occurs at roughly the same pace as the decomposition of existing bone. Accordingly, the adult skeleton undergoes a complete renewal process over 7–10 years.

After age 40, the bone starts to break down more quickly than it is rebuilt, which causes our bones to gradually lose density. As we age, we all experience some bone loss, but osteoporosis is only referred to when the bones become extremely brittle.

A bone damaged by osteoporosis has greater pores in the honeycomb structure and a reduced overall density, which increases the risk of fracture. A medical disease called osteoporosis weakens bones, making them brittle and more prone to shatter. It takes years to grow slowly and is sometimes only discovered when a bone breaks (fractures) due to trauma from a fall or other rapid impact.

When someone has osteoporosis, the following injuries are most typical:

- Sprained wrist
- Fractured hip (broken hip)
- Fractured vertebrae in the spine

But other bones, such as those in the arm or pelvis, can also shatter. A cough or sneeze may occasionally result in a cracked rib or the partial collapse of one of the spine's bones. Osteoporosis often does not produce pain until a bone is shattered, although damaged spines are a major source of chronic pain.

Even though a fractured bone is frequently the initial indication of osteoporosis, some elderly individuals have the recognizable stooped (bent forward) posture. It occurs when the spine's bones are shattered, making it difficult for the body to sustain its weight.

Symptoms

Osteoporosis usually does not have symptoms. The first indication that you could have it is when you have a low-impact fracture, which is when a bone is broken in a relatively modest fall or accident. The hip, spine, or wrist are the most frequent places for fractures.

Some people experience back issues if their vertebrae, or spine's bones, weaken and shorten. Vertebral crush fractures are what they are called. They often occur in the middle or lower back and can take place without any injuries.

Your spine will start to bend if many vertebrae are injured, and you might get shorter as a result. Because there is less room behind the ribs, breathing can occasionally become problematic after spinal crush fractures. You have a higher chance of breaking your wrists or hips if you have a spinal crush fracture.

The Causes and Risk Factors of Osteoporosis

An unbalanced ratio of new bone production to old bone resorption leads to osteoporosis. Osteoclasts demolish bone tissues during bone resorption, releasing specific minerals that move calcium from the bone to the blood. With osteoporosis, the body may not produce enough new bone or absorb too much of the existing bone.

The possibility of both outcomes exists as well. Osteoporosis typically takes several years to develop after bone loss. Most of the time, it takes suffering a fracture for a person to realize they have the disorder.

The disease will have advanced by then, and the harm it causes may be extremely severe. Age, gender, hormones, using particular drugs, and having specific medical conditions are some of the most typical risk factors and causes of osteoporosis.

Age

Osteoporosis primarily develops as a result of aging. Your skeleton starts to lose more bone as you age than it gains. Additionally, the solid outer covering of bones becomes thinner while the microscopic holes inside them begin to become larger. Your bones are less thick as a result. Hard bones become pliable, while pliable bones become even pliable.

Osteoporosis develops when bone density loss reaches a particular threshold. Insufficient bone density makes bones more brittle and less able to withstand falls. The majority of specialists advise beginning osteoporosis screening around age 65, particularly for women, although those who are at high risk for fractures should begin screening sooner.

Menopause, low estrogen, and gender

Women often have smaller, thinner bones than males, which is one of the major causes of the greater risk. Another factor is the significant decline in estrogen levels that occurs when a woman enters menopause.

Estrogen is the hormone in women that protects bones. Reduced bone density is a recognized result of the absence of estrogen, which is a normal side effect of menopause. In reaction to the drastic drop in estrogen levels, a woman enters menopause at which time she stops ovulating and ceases having monthly periods. A woman's bone density will decline the longer her levels are low.

The following are additional elements that raise a woman's risk for osteoporosis:
- Early Menopause – Before the age of 45.
- Enduring a prolonged stretch of menstruation.
- Irregular menstrual cycles, a sign that a lady is not ovulating adequately.

Reduced testosterone

Men with hypogonadism, or low testosterone levels, frequently develop osteoporosis. Low testosterone levels cause the loss of bone density over time, which finally results in weak bones that are brittle and prone to fractures from little stress.

Medications

The chance of developing osteoporosis can rise when certain drugs, such as long-term oral and injectable corticosteroids, are used. Corticosteroid drugs have the potential to weaken a person's bones when taken for longer durations and at larger doses.

Osteoporosis can also be brought on by thyroid medicines, SSRIs, chemotherapy treatments, and other medications. Of course, these drugs may be vital for treating a variety of ailments. As a result, you should always consult your healthcare practitioner before stopping any therapy or changing your dosage.

Some Medical Conditions

Bone loss is a side effect of certain common medical diseases. You are more likely to get osteoporosis if you have one of these illnesses. Secondary osteoporosis is osteoporosis that is brought on by another illness.

Diabetes, autoimmune inflammatory illnesses, thyroid issues, and malabsorption syndromes are all factors connected to osteoporosis.

According to several research, patients with type 1 diabetes arc likely to have lower bone density than average. They may also have slower bone turnover and less bone growth.

The body assaults its healthy tissues in inflammatory autoimmune disorders like rheumatoid arthritis and lupus, which result in widespread systemic inflammation. It is thought that inflammatory conditions raise the likelihood of bone turnover. Corticosteroids, a common cause of osteoporosis since they may slow down the activities of bone-building cells, are also used by people with these diseases.

Bone Density

The most significant indicator of risk for osteoporosis is typically bone mass. By the time they reach their late 20s, most people have reached their peak bone mass or the largest bone mass they are capable of reaching.

Genetics also determines peak bone mass. People who are genetically predisposed to the illness and have a family history of it will peak in bone mass considerably sooner.

Bone mass is also influenced by family history; if your parents had healthy bones, there is a greater likelihood that you will as well.

Genetic Propensity

Certain people have a significant hereditary predisposition to osteoporosis. In actuality, a person might inherit many genes that raise their risk of getting the illness.

Behavioral Risk Factors

Numerous osteoporosis risk factors may be beyond your control.

However, several risk factors related to your lifestyle that are under your control may also increase your risk.

Not getting enough calcium and vitamin D

Because calcium and vitamin D operate in tandem to support bone health, it is crucial to have a diet rich in both of these minerals.

Calcium promotes strong bones, and vitamin D makes it easier for the body to absorb calcium.

A Sedentary Way of Life

Exercise prevents osteoporosis and maintains the strength of the bones and muscles. Strong bones also have a lower chance of breaking.

Smoking

Smoking and reduced bone mass are correlated directly. This link exists for several reasons. First, the chemicals in cigarettes can disrupt the normal operation of the cells in your bones.

Smoking can inhibit the absorption of calcium. Additionally, it may lessen the bone-protective effects of estrogen. According to studies, smoking increases the risk of fractures and might delay the healing of existing fractures.

Alcohol Overconsumption

Alcohol consumption has a detrimental impact on bone health. One of the causes is that it disrupts the body's calcium balance and vitamin D absorption.

Hormone deficits can also result from excessive drinking in both men and women. The bone-forming cells called osteoblasts may potentially be killed by excessive alcohol use. Alcohol misuse can also alter balance and gait, which can result in falls that frequently cause fractures owing to fragile bones and nerve damage.

How Osteoporosis Affects the Body

The condition of osteoporosis damages the body's bones. Loss of bone density, which renders the bones brittle and more prone to fractures, is one of its defining characteristics.

Although any bone in the body can be affected by this illness, the wrists, hips, and spine are the most frequently affected. Our bodies regularly break down and rebuild the living tissue that makes up our bones. Our bodies can repair bones more quickly while we are young than they can break them down, which enables our bones to develop and strengthen.

However, this process slows down and our bones start to lose density as we become older. Osteoporosis patients experience a decrease in bone density because the rate of bone deterioration outpaces the rate of bone regrowth. Fractures are more likely as a result of the bones being weaker and more brittle.

Back discomfort is one of the most prevalent signs of osteoporosis and may be brought on by fractures in the spine's vertebrae. Even slight trauma, such as bending over or carrying anything heavy, can result in these fractures.

Serious instances might result in the vertebrae collapsing, which can reduce the height and result in a stooped posture. Other bones, such as the hips and wrists, can also break due to osteoporosis. These fractures could be excruciatingly painful, and they might take a while to heal. They may even result in long-term incapacity in rare circumstances.

Osteoporosis can have various effects on the body besides fractures. For instance, it may result in a loss of freedom and movement as well as a higher risk of depression and other mental health problems. Osteoporosis is often treated with a cocktail of drugs, dietary modifications, and physical therapy.

The pace of bone loss can be slowed down and the rate of bone regrowth can be accelerated with the use of medications. A balanced diet and regular exercise are other good ways to enhance bone density and lower the risk of fractures.

In summary, osteoporosis is a disease that affects the body's bones, resulting in a decrease in bone density and a higher risk of fractures. Back discomfort, hip and wrist fractures, as well as a reduction in mobility and independence, can all result from it. Physical therapy, dietary modifications, and pharmaceuticals are frequently used in conjunction with treatment.

CHAPTER TWO: DIAGNOSIS AND TESTING

How Osteoporosis is Diagnosed

Osteoporosis diagnosis often involves many processes. A doctor will carefully assess both your osteoporosis and fracture risks. Following are the steps for diagnosing osteoporosis:

Gathering health history

The risk factors for osteoporosis will be the subject of a doctor's inquiry. Your risk rises if you have a family history of osteoporosis. Your risk may also be impacted by lifestyle variables including food, exercise, alcohol use, and smoking.

Your medical history will be discussed with a doctor, along with any drugs you may have taken. Your doctor may inquire about your history of back discomfort, any recent bone fractures, any height loss over time, or stooped posture if you exhibit any of the symptoms of osteoporosis.

Taking a physical examination

A physician will gauge a patient's height and compare it to earlier readings. Loss in height may be a sign of osteoporosis. If you have trouble getting up from a seated posture without using your arms to lift yourself, your doctor might inquire.

Additionally, they could do some other blood tests to assess your vitamin D levels and the general metabolic activity of your bones. Osteoporosis may increase metabolic activity.

Having a bone density test done

A bone density test may be required if a doctor finds that you are at risk for osteoporosis. A dual-energy X-ray absorptiometry (DEXA) scan is a typical illustration. X-ray pictures are used in this quick, painless procedure to assess fracture risk and bone density.

Carrying out blood and urine tests

Bone loss can be brought on by medical issues. These include thyroid and parathyroid issues. To rule this out, a doctor could do blood and urine tests. Men's testosterone levels, thyroid function, and calcium levels may all be tested.

Mineral Density of Bone

Doctors will probably request a bone density scan to identify osteoporosis, evaluate the risk of bone fracture, and decide the best course of therapy. Bone mineral density is measured with this scan.

Dual-energy X-ray absorptiometry (DXA) is frequently used in its execution. The amount of X-rays that are absorbed by tissues and bone is measured by the DXA equipment and is connected to bone mineral density. Bone density data is converted into T- and Z-scores using the DXA equipment. The T-score calculates how much bone you have in comparison to a population of 30-year-olds.

This T-score is used to determine if medication therapy is necessary as well as the likelihood of getting a fracture. Regarding the T-score, a score of > -1 indicates normal bone density and a score of -2.5 indicates a greater risk of osteoporosis. When compared to people of the same age and sex, your Z-score indicates how much bone you have.

FRAX Rating

Doctors have created a tool called the Fracture Risk Assessment Tool, or FRAX, to assess the risk of damage. This calculates your likelihood of suffering a hip fracture or other significant fracture in the following ten years. A healthcare professional often administers the FRAX, which entails answering numerous questions about your lifestyle choices, including your alcohol consumption and other conditions that may be connected to osteoporosis.

Your FRAX scores are computed by the program as you enter this data. It's crucial to understand your 10-year fracture risk since it will help you choose your therapy more carefully. You may be at an elevated risk of fractures if your FRAX score is 20% or more for severe osteoporosis fractures or 3% or more for hip fractures.

The Importance of Early Diagnosis

Osteoporosis is typically detected in people who have fractures or other bone deterioration because of the condition's basic nature. The greatest method to prevent this and lessen the pain of those affected is early screening. Nobody enters their doctor's office declaring, "I think I have osteoporosis." The majority of people don't even realize they have the problem until they go to the doctor for a fractured bone, a vertebra, or something much worse.

The disease is only then thereafter diagnosed. Because of this, it's critical to control and relieve the effects of osteoporosis as soon as feasible. From a financial standpoint, this is crucial since it stops the progression of osteoporosis, which means patients won't sustain more broken, shattered, or crushed bones. Because it can stop or halt the growth of the ailment, early detection of osteoporosis is crucial.

Early detection of osteoporosis allows for the initiation of treatment to assist maintain or increase bone density, which can lower the risk of fractures. Additionally, early diagnosis can assist in determining any underlying medical issues that might be influencing the onset of osteoporosis. For instance, osteoporosis can be exacerbated by certain drugs and medical conditions, therefore recognizing these causes early on might assist to stop the disease from progressing.

Any lifestyle variables that could be causing osteoporosis to develop might be found with an early diagnosis. Making dietary adjustments early on can help to prevent the illness from growing worse since eating a diet low in calcium and vitamin D can raise the risk of osteoporosis. Last but not least, early diagnosis might enhance the quality of life.

Early treatment of osteoporosis can help to lessen its symptoms and enhance the overall quality of life because it can lead to pain, incapacity, and a loss of independence. The early detection of osteoporosis is crucial because it can assist to stop or delay the condition's progression, uncover any underlying medical conditions or lifestyle concerns, and enhance the quality of life.

CHAPTER THREE: TREATMENT AND MANAGEMENT

Medications for Osteoporosis

Treatment options for osteoporosis (and occasionally osteopenia) span a wide range of medications.

Bisphosphonates

The rate at which your body breaks down bone is slowed by bisphosphonates. By doing this, you preserve bone density and lower your chance of breaking a bone. Numerous distinct bisphosphonates exist, including:

- Alendronic acid
- Ibandronic acid
- Zoledronic acid
- Risedronate

They can be administered as a tablet, a liquid to be ingested, or an injection.

Always consume a full glass of water along with bisphosphonates on an empty stomach. After taking these, stay upright for 30 minutes.

Additionally, you must wait anywhere from 30 minutes to 2 hours before eating or drinking anything else. You may need to take bisphosphonates for up to five years before they start to work, which typically takes six to twelve months.

Additionally, you can be given calcium and vitamin D supplements to take separately from the bisphosphonate. The primary negative effects of bisphosphonates include swallowing issues, food pipe irritation, and abdominal pain.

Although it occurs more commonly with high-dose intravenous bisphosphonate therapy for cancer rather than osteoporosis, osteonecrosis of the jaw is an uncommon adverse effect associated with the use of bisphosphonates.

In osteonecrosis, the jaw bone's cells start to die, which can cause issues with healing. Before beginning bisphosphonate therapy, you may require a checkup if you have a history of dental issues. Whenever you have any worries, talk to your doctor.

Selective Estrogen Receptor Modulators (SERMs)
SERMs are drugs with effects on bone that are comparable to those of estrogen. They contribute to maintaining bone density and lowering fracture risk, particularly for the spine. The only SERM available for the treatment of osteoporosis is raloxifene. Only women are advised to use it after menopause. It is taken as a pill every day. There are several raloxifene side effects which includes leg

cramps, hot flashes, and a possible rise in blood clot risk.

Thyroid hormone

The body naturally produces the hormone parathyroid. It controls the calcium content in bones. Cells that form new bones are stimulated by parathyroid hormone therapies (such as teriparatide). Once a day, you receive an injection of these.

Parathyroid hormone can boost bone density whilst other medications can simply decrease the pace of bone weakening. However, it's only applied to a limited percentage of patients with extremely low bone densities and when conventional therapies are failing.

Dizziness, headaches, and nausea are frequent adverse effects of the therapy.

Biomedical remedies

Biomedical drugs are created using the body's proteins or other materials. Denosumab and romosozumab are biological medications that can be used to treat osteoporosis. They could be suggested if you have severe osteoporosis or can't take other medications like bisphosphonates.

They function by increasing the pace at which your cells make new bones while decreasing the rate at which your bones are broken down. Every month or every several months, they are injected. Muscle or joint discomfort, rashes, constipation, and cold-like sensations are typical adverse effects.

Vitamin D and Calcium supplements

The primary mineral present in bones is calcium, thus eating a diet high in calcium as part of a healthy, balanced diet is crucial for keeping strong bones. The recommended daily calcium intake for most healthy individuals is 700 milligrams (mg), which most people should be able to obtain via a diversified diet that includes calcium-rich foods.

Hormone Replacement Therapy

Women going through menopause can utilize HRT (hormone replacement therapy) to assist manage symptoms. HRT has also been demonstrated to maintain bone density and lower the chance of developing osteoporosis. It can strengthen your bones and lower your chance of fracturing a bone if you already have osteoporosis.

You will typically be recommended to use HRT or hormonal contraception until at least age 51 if you have early menopause, in which case your periods cease before the age of 45. This raises your estrogen levels, assisting in your defense against osteoporosis and other illnesses.

The risk of breast cancer is modestly increased by several HRT forms. Long-term HRT use puts you in greater danger. The chance of blood clots is somewhat increased by HRT pills, but not by patches, gel, or spray. Your age, symptoms, and other risk factors you may have will determine if HRT is the correct choice for you. The advantages of HRT often outweigh the hazards if you're under 60 and experiencing menopausal symptoms.

Lifestyle Changes for Osteoporosis

Lifestyle changes can be very helpful in both treating and preventing osteoporosis. Following are some lifestyle modifications that might enhance bone health:

Exercise often.
Exercise can lower the incidence of falls and fractures by enhancing balance and coordination. Weight-bearing exercise promotes bone density and enhances balance, hence lowering the risk of falls.

Osteoporosis that is already advanced is not treated. Before beginning a new fitness regimen, speak with your doctor, especially if you have been inactive, are older than 75, or have a medical problem. Some general suggestions are:

- Pick weight-bearing exercises like jogging, brisk walking, tennis, netball, or dancing. Swimming and cycling are great non-weight-bearing workouts for numerous health reasons, but they do not stimulate bone formation.
- Jumping and rope skipping are two exercises with a strong impact that you should incorporate into your program. Consult a health specialist before beginning any high-impact fitness program if you suffer from joint issues, another medical condition, or are physically unfit.
- Another crucial activity for bone health is strength training (also known as resistance

training). In order to grow and sustain muscular strength, muscular endurance, and muscular mass, resistance must be given to a muscle. Strength training is crucial for maintaining or even increasing bone mineral density, which is important for managing and preventing osteoporosis. Follow the advice of a fitness or health expert (such as an exercise physiologist), who may suggest certain workouts and methods.

- Exercises that improve muscular strength, balance, and coordination, like tai chi, Pilates, and mild yoga, are particularly crucial since they can lower your risk of falling by enhancing your posture, balance, and muscle strength. It is best to spread out your strength-training and weight-bearing workouts throughout the week. Four to six times each week, aim for 30 to 40 minutes. Regular and varied exercise is necessary for bone formation.

Eat a balanced diet.

Bone health depends on consuming a diet high in calcium and vitamin D. Dairy products, leafy green vegetables, and fortified meals are all excellent sources of calcium. Sunlight, vitamins, and certain meals like fatty fish and fortified foods can all help you get enough vitamin D.

Building and keeping strong, healthy bones requires eating a healthy, balanced diet that includes a variety of foods and getting enough calcium. Your body will remove calcium from your bones if there is not enough calcium in the blood. Getting adequate calcium via your diet is crucial for maintaining bone density.

The largest calcium content is found in dairy products, but there are several additional calcium-rich foods, such as sardines, spinach, and almonds. You might need to discuss calcium supplements with a healthcare provider if your diet isn't providing you with enough calcium on its own. Bone density is enhanced by calcium and vitamin D. Because it facilitates the body's absorption of the calcium in your diet, vitamin D is crucial.

Additionally, foods like fatty fish (salmon, herring, and mackerel), liver, eggs, and fortified foods like low-fat milk and margarine contain vitamin D in trace amounts.

It is doubtful that most individuals will be able to get enough vitamin D through food alone. If you are worried that you are not receiving enough vitamin D, talk to your healthcare provider about vitamin D supplements.

Stop smoking.
Smoking has been associated with an increased incidence of bone fractures and osteoporosis.

Giving up smoking can help strengthen bones and lower the risk of fractures.

Limit your alcohol intake.

The risk of bone loss and fractures might rise with excessive alcohol use. One drink a day is the maximum amount that should be consumed to maintain bone health. If you do consume alcohol, do it in moderation since too much of it raises the risk of osteoporosis. Have no more than two standard drinks per day and at least two days per week without alcohol.

Decrease the chance of falls

By taking precautions to lower the risk of falls, fractures can be avoided. This might involve eliminating trip risks from the home, donning the proper footwear, and utilizing aids like canes or walkers. Every year, a third of persons over the age of 65 falls, and 6% of those falls result in a fracture. The danger of falls must be decreased.

Be led by your physician, but here are some broad suggestions:

- Follow the training regimen recommended by a physiotherapist or exercise physiologist to enhance your balance.
- If you wear prescription glasses, do so by your eye doctor's instructions.
- Make your home "trip proof" by, for instance, taking out any loose rugs, adding handrails to the shower and the toilet, and making sure all areas are properly lighted. This is where an occupational therapist may assist.
- Put on dependable flat-heeled footwear that fits well.
- Think about donning a hip protector. This shield, which is worn over the hip, is intended to disperse the force of a fall away from the hipbone and towards the nearby fat

and muscle. A hip protector worn properly can lower the risk of hip fracture.

Keep your body at a healthy weight.
Osteoporosis and fracture risk might rise with underweight status. Bone health can be enhanced by maintaining healthy body weight through a balanced diet and frequent exercise.

In conclusion, modifying one's lifestyle may be very helpful in both treating and preventing osteoporosis. Bone health may be enhanced by engaging in regular exercise, eating a good diet, stopping smoking, consuming alcohol in moderation, lowering the risk of falls, and keeping a healthy body weight.

CHAPTER FOUR: COMPLICATIONS AND PREVENTION

Common Complications of Osteoporosis

Osteoporosis can result in several problems, such as:

Fractures

There's not much keeping your bones from abruptly shattering as they deteriorate. They no longer possess the strength and flexibility that allowed them to withstand great stress. Even the smallest mistake, such as a simple stumble, might cause a shattered bone.

The most common sites for osteoporosis-related fractures are high-impact, load-bearing structures like your hip, wrist, and spine. The most frequent side effect of osteoporosis is fractures. Because osteoporosis weakens bones, they are more prone to breaking. Hip, spine, and wrist fractures are all possible, and they can cause discomfort, impairment, and loss of freedom.

A particularly significant side effect of osteoporosis is hip fractures. They can result in severe discomfort and incapacity, as well as a loss of independence and a worse quality of life. Especially for older persons, hip fractures are linked to an increased risk of death.

Another frequent consequence of osteoporosis is spinal fractures. They may result in persistent discomfort, height reduction, and hunched posture. In addition to compressing the spinal nerves, spinal fractures can cause weakness, tingling, and numbness in the arms and legs.

Additionally, wrist fractures are more frequent in those with osteoporosis. They may result in edema, discomfort, and restricted range of motion in the wrist and hand. An essential component of controlling osteoporosis is preventing fractures.

This might involve engaging in regular physical activity, maintaining a nutritious diet, stopping smoking, using alcohol in moderation, and taking medicines as directed by a doctor.

Additionally, it's critical to take precautions to lessen the chance of falls by doing things like clearing the house of any tripping hazards, using the proper footwear, and employing aids like walkers or canes.

Pain

There are several causes of pain, ranging from an inflamed nerve to a painful muscle, for instance. However, if you have osteoporosis, your discomfort is caused by a shattered bone. Even a little fracture may be excruciatingly painful.

You might not be aware that your discomfort is coming from a fracture because it can occur at any time. Chronic pain can be brought on by fractures and bone loss, which can be difficult to manage and lower quality of life. Any area of the body afflicted by osteoporosis might experience chronic pain, although the wrists, hips, and back are the most often impacted.

Pain can be either regular or sporadic, intense, dull, or agonizing. Life may be significantly impacted by pain. Daily tasks like getting dressed, cooking, or cleaning up might become challenging. Additionally, it can disrupt sleep, which results in weariness and a worse quality of life. It might be difficult to manage osteoporosis-related chronic discomfort.

Nonsteroidal anti-inflammatory medicines (NSAIDs) and opioid painkillers may be beneficial, but they can have negative side effects and may not work for all types of pain. For the treatment of chronic pain, physical therapy, acupuncture, and other alternative therapies may also be beneficial.

An essential aspect of treating the chronic pain brought on by osteoporosis is preventing fractures. This might involve engaging in regular physical activity, maintaining a nutritious diet, stopping smoking, using alcohol in moderation, and taking medicines as directed by a doctor.

Additionally, it's critical to take precautions to lessen the chance of falls by doing things like clearing the house of any tripping hazards, using the proper footwear, and employing aids like walkers or canes.

Decline in height

Your spine contributes significantly to your stature. Osteoporosis can cause the vertebrae in the spine to collapse as it steadily erodes your bones and weakens your vertebrae, resulting in a loss of height and a hunched posture. You'll see that you've become shorter by one or two inches.

Reduced mobility

Osteoporosis frequently leads to complications including restricted movement. Losing mobility due to osteoporosis can be difficult to manage and can lower quality of life. Any area of the body affected by osteoporosis might experience decreased mobility, but the wrists, hips, and back are most susceptible to it.

Walking, getting dressed, and carrying out domestic chores may be challenging when there are fractures in these locations. Losing movement can have a big effect on day-to-day living. It may result in diminished quality of life, social isolation, and a loss of independence.

Depression
Numerous factors including osteoporosis can contribute to depression. Depression can be exacerbated by osteoporosis-related chronic pain, impairment, and mobility loss. Depression may also

be exacerbated by the social isolation that might follow a loss of mobility.

Osteoporosis frequently exhibits symptoms of chronic discomfort. Debilitating pain can make it difficult to carry out everyday tasks, which can cause irritation, worry, and sadness. Additionally, the pain might make it difficult to fall asleep, which can worsen sadness.

Depression may also be exacerbated by osteoporosis-related impairment and decreased mobility. It can be challenging to cope with losing one's freedom and the capacity to engage in things that one formerly liked. In addition, maintaining a chronic disease can be extremely stressful and exacerbate depression.

Depression can also be exacerbated by social isolation. It may be challenging to leave the house and engage in social activities if you lose your mobility. This may result in feelings of isolation and loneliness, which may fuel depression.

Increased mortality risk
Numerous factors, including osteoporosis, can raise the chance of death. The most typical method involves fractures. In older people, fractures can set off a series of circumstances that could finally result in mortality.

Significant pain and suffering brought on by fractures may result in loss of independence and movement. This may result in a lower quality of life and a higher chance of developing depression and other mental health problems.

Complications from fractures might include blood clots, pneumonia, and infections. These problems can be fatal, especially in elderly people who may already be suffering from underlying medical disorders. Additionally, muscular mass and strength loss brought on by fractures might raise the likelihood of falls and fractures. This may set off a vicious cycle that eventually results in a lower standard of living and a higher risk of death.

Osteoporosis Prevention Strategies

Here are prevention strategies for osteoporosis:

1. Get adequate vitamin D and calcium.
2. Regularly do weight-bearing exercise.
3. Give up smoking.
4. Drink with moderation.
5. Avoid consuming too much caffeine.
6. Consume a diet high in fruits and vegetables to stay healthy.
7. Keep your weight within a healthy range.
8. Discuss your risk of osteoporosis with your healthcare professional.
9. Take a look at bone density testing.

10. As directed by your healthcare practitioner, take medicine.

11. Avoid falling and take precautions to avoid it.

12. Use assistance aids if necessary and dress appropriately for the weather.

13. Your home's lighting can be improved to lower the danger of falls.

14. Eliminate trip risks from your house.

15. Keep moving to keep your muscles flexible and strong.

16. If you have osteoporosis, stay away from high-impact sports.

17. If neccssary, take into account hormone replacement treatment (HRT).

18. When using specific drugs that might raise the risk of osteoporosis, use care.

19. Think about alternative treatments like massage or acupuncture.

20. Develop a thorough treatment plan that addresses your unique requirements in

collaboration with your healthcare practitioner.

21. Sleep enough to aid in your body's regrowth.

22. Through yoga, meditation, or other practices, you can lower your tension and anxiety.

23. Install handrails and remove tripping hazards among other fall prevention measures.

24. Whenever necessary, use aids like canes or walkers.

25. Exercises for building strength and balance can be done.

26. Steer clear of smoking and passive smoking.

27. Drink with moderation.

28. Any drugs that might make you more susceptible to osteoporosis should be discussed with your healthcare professional.

29. Think about taking calcium, vitamin D, and magnesium supplements.

30. Keep up with the latest findings and therapies for osteoporosis.

31. Limit your intake of vitamin A.

32. Eat less sugar and processed food.

33. Avoid consuming soda and other drinks with added sugar.

34. Consume omega-3 fatty acid-rich meals.

35. Aim to limit your salt intake.

36. Obtain enough vitamin K.

37. Install grab bars in the bathroom, for instance, to prevent falls at home.

38. Put on supportive footwear with non-slip soles.

39. Spend as little time as possible sitting still.

40. If you are not receiving enough calcium from your diet, think about taking a calcium supplement.

Keep in mind that the best defense against osteoporosis is prevention. You can lower your chance of getting this illness by taking actions to maintain strong bones.

CHAPTER FIVE: LIVING WITH OSTEOPOROSIS

How to talk to your Doctor about Osteoporosis

Discussing osteoporosis with your doctor can be a crucial first step in treating your disease and lowering your risk of problems.

You've decided to discuss osteoporosis with your doctor. Perhaps you are now worried that you might forget to ask all the questions you need to ask the doctor during your appointment or that you could forget to mention something during your visit. The following advice will help you be ready for your appointment and make the most of your doctor's time.

Get Ready for the Visit

1. Your medical history is essential, but so is the medical history of your family. Tell your

doctor, for instance, if your mother has or has ever had osteoporosis.

2. Tell your doctor right away if you have hyperthyroidism (overactive thyroid), lung issues, kidney or liver illness, multiple sclerosis, rheumatoid arthritis, or any other medical conditions.

3. Review the osteoporosis risk factors for a short while. Make a list of the hazards that concern you.

4. Make a list of all the prescription and over-the-counter medications you use. Add supplements or vitamins. Add these to your list if you have had treatment for cancer, an endocrine disorder (such as a thyroid issue), epilepsy, or menopause (hormone replacement therapy).

5. Have you ever had corticosteroid spinal injections to treat back pain? If so, remember to record this.

Questions to Ask

1. I either get rapid onset of back pain or persistent back pain. Is an X-ray necessary?
2. Should I be tested for bone density? Please explain this test to me.
3. Describe the T-score. How would you rate me? When should the bone density test be repeated?
4. Do my drugs make me more likely to develop osteoporosis?
5. How much exercise do I need to perform to strengthen my bones?
6. Is using hormone replacement therapy to ward against osteoporosis safe?
7. I find it challenging to begin and maintain an exercise routine. Please assist me.
8. I want to cut back or stop smoking. Please assist me.
9. What treatments are available to manage osteoporosis if I have it?

10. Should I be aware of anything else concerning osteoporosis?

What the Doctor Might Ask You

1. Which prescription drugs do you use, and why?
2. Does your back hurt?
3. Have your joints or bones ever hurt or felt uncomfortable?
4. What is the duration of your back pain?
5. Have you ever shattered a bone or suffered from a fracture?
6. Have you lately been injured?
7. When was the last time you had your vision examined?
8. Have you had any further medical diagnoses made?
9. Do you ever become lightheaded or woozy?
10. Is there a history of osteoporosis in the family?
11. Are you a smoker?

12. Are you an alcoholic? If so, how much and how frequently?

13. What meals do you consume?

14. Do you regularly diet?

15. Do you work out? Which kind of exercise, and how frequently?

16. Have your posture or height changed over time?

17. Do you now use any vitamins or supplements?

18. Have you ever had osteoporosis treatment?

19. Do you have any worries or queries regarding your health or available treatments?

You may control your osteoporosis and lower your risk of consequences by being an active participant in your healthcare and collaborating closely with your doctor.

CONCLUSION

The Future of Osteoporosis Prevention and Treatment

With constant research and technological developments producing fresh and creative ideas, the future of osteoporosis prevention and treatment is bright. The creation of novel drugs to treat osteoporosis is one field of study.

Although there are already many effective drugs accessible, they frequently have drawbacks and adverse effects. To boost bone formation while avoiding side effects on other bodily systems, researchers are looking into novel medications that can target particular bone cells.

The enhancement of bone health by dietary and nutritional changes is the subject of more investigation. A diet high in calcium, vitamin D, and other minerals has been demonstrated in studies to maintain bone health and lower the incidence of osteoporosis.

Researchers are looking for novel ways to provide essential nutrients in the diet, such as supplements or fortified foods. Technology advancements are also influencing how osteoporosis will be prevented and treated in the future.

For instance, wearable technology and sensors can support tracking long-term changes in bone density and monitoring it. This enables medical professionals to recognize early osteoporosis symptoms and create specialized treatment regimens.

New fitness programs and physical rehabilitation procedures are also being developed using virtual reality and other technology. These programs are more efficient and practical than conventional fitness programs since they can be customized to meet individual requirements and abilities.

Overall, there is hope for the future of osteoporosis prevention and treatment because of continuous research and technological breakthroughs that are producing fresh ideas.

We can enhance bone health and lessen the effects of osteoporosis on individuals and society at large by continuing to invest in research and technology.

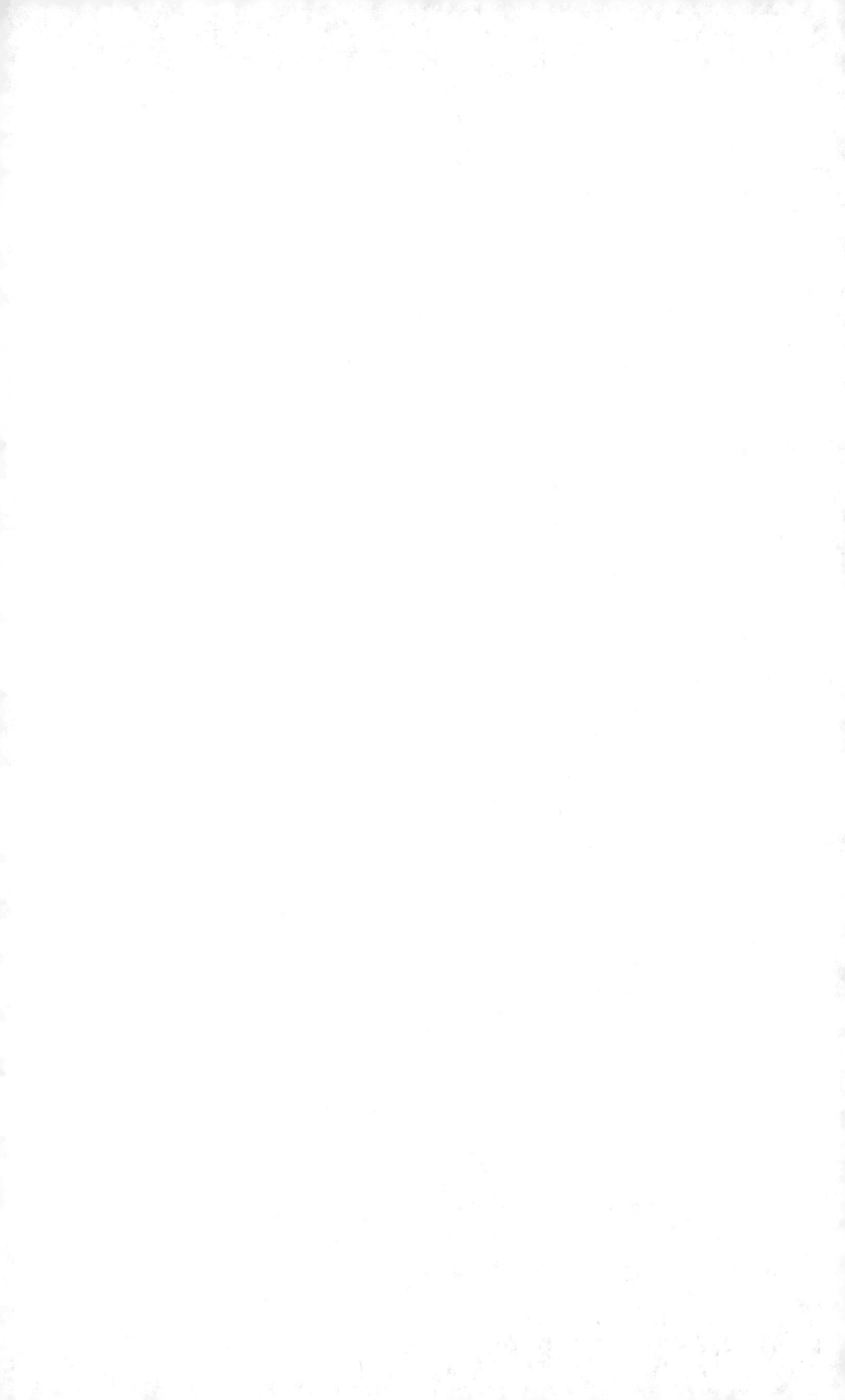